THE IMMUNE SYSTEM HEALTH GUIDEBOOK

Paul Schulick

ISBN 0-937643-00-9

Library of Congress 86-080647

Edited by Barbara Landgarten Schulick

Published by:

**Herbal Formula Research
PO Box 1947
Brattleboro, VT   05301**

Manufactured by Apollo Books, 107 Lafayette St., Winona, MN 55987

PRINTED IN THE UNITED STATES OF AMERICA

TABLE OF CONTENTS

It is traditional for an author like myself to preface a guidebook like this with a disclaimer. It helps protect you the reader from unprofessional advice and myself the author from misrepresentation. I make it very clear to all to whom I lecture or counsel that I am not a doctor. The advice that I give should not be misconstrued as a prescription or as a replacement for the care of a doctor. There is, however, a Catch-22 inherent in these disclaimers. All the disclaimers advise getting medical attention, yet the people who offer the medical care are often in direct conflict with the very principles the books are suggesting. Also when the disclaimers are routinely declared, it inevitably tends to sound like a disavowal of important information. Where does this leave the reader? The seeker of health is left in a state of deeper confusion and with a lack of direction. What is the solution? The luminaries in medicine and science need to apply their skills to unite natural healing principles like the ones offered in this guidebook with the strict standards of modern science. Instead of routinely criticizing age-old remedies as unproven and excluding many valuable therapeutics, some of the vast resources available to modern research should be spent to "scientifically" separate the useful from the useless. Surely there is enough evidence to stimulate this type of inquiry. Especially now that we can see the shortcomings or failures of such highly touted modern techniques like bypasses, chemotherapy and mammary amputations, it is clear that there is room for thorough investigations of nature's potential healing tools. With this more complete understanding, societal health would take a quantum leap. With this in mind, please accept the scientific information offered in this guidebook as suggestive, but unfortunately not yet proven. Urge your dedicated physician to read this guidebook and the references cited and suggest the idea of cooperation. Study and work with your doctor to create optimal health.

INTRODUCTION

In our recent times, there is rarely a day that goes by in which the immune or disease defense system does not make front page headlines. Unfortunately these days it is all in terms of the horrific disease AIDS (Acquired Immune Deficiency Syndrome). Those suffering from this disease see a gradual degeneration of their usual immune system responses and eventually die of cancer or infection. Besides forcing us to reflect upon our personal lifestyles, AIDS has stimulated a deeper appreciation and concern for the health of our immune system. We are becoming aware that everything from cancer and heart disease to the ubiquitous "cold" falls under the influence of this important body system. We know that if the system is in harmony and is strong, there is evidence that these conditions will be less lethal or prevented, and when the system is imbalanced and weak, the worst cases are realized. Recognizing the vital role our immune system can play, one noted scientist said, "Every week we may get cancer. And every week we may reject it."

Fortunately, there are health support guidelines for the immune system. Contrary to what many standard health care practitioners may say or suggest, the immune system can be cared for. Like all other body organs, the group of tissues responsible for what we call the immune response are subject to variable degrees of stress. Innumerable scientific studies have confirmed that these stresses can severely affect immune system strength. Fortunately or unfortunately many of these stresses are under our voluntary control. It is often our choice whether we abuse and hastily wear down the system or nurture and regenerate it. If we can learn more about these choices and how to modify them in our favor, then the goal of a stronger immune system can be achieved.

By taking one example of when the immune system is traditionally weakest, we can discover many of the influences which can shape its strength. The changing seasons, particularly the first cold winds of winter, represent a time of test for the immune system. It is during this time that we are either most concerned about or experience our once or twice a year cold or infection. We will see through our analysis of winter that the health of the immune system is not as whimsical as is commonly believed, and that there are choices we can make and tools we can use which will better our state of immunity and our prospects for long-term vitality.

A DEFINITION

The immune system is an intricate biochemical complex which allows the body to protect itself against malignancies, foreign bodies and pathogenic organisms. Malignancies are cancers or foreign cell masses, which through their uncontrolled growth, compete and interfere with normal cell metabolism. Foreign bodies can be everything from a microscopic ragweed seed to an internally produced metabolic by-product like incomplete protein breakdown substances (IPBs). Pathogenic organisms range from the common cold virus and ubiquitous candida albicans fungi to Clostridium botulinum and the AIDS producing virus. Whatever the invading organism though, it should be clear that when the immune system is weak, the common cold virus or ragweed can become as deadly as the AIDS virus HTLV 111.

The mechanical effectiveness of the immune system is principally determined by the success of two distinct responses called the humoral and cell-mediated response. The humoral response is the immune system's generation of B-cells which produce antibodies that react with or neutralize foreign bodies. The cell-mediated response is the term given for the immune system's creation of T-cells which mobilize and stimulate "attack" cells called phagocytes to engulf and digest invading microorganisms. Coordinated with these two interdependent activities, the immune system also protects the body from infection by stimulating the inflammatory and fever process and creating protective blood proteins like interferon. We are all gifted with a genetically active immune system and an acquired immune response. This means that part of our immunity is gained through inheritance and the rest is obtained through accumulated responses to foreign body exposures. The principal organs of the immune system are the thymus, bone marrow, spleen, and lymphoid tissues like the tonsils in the throat and the Peyer's patches in the intestines.

Balance or homeostasis is a key word in evaluating the effectiveness of immune system functioning. When homeostasis of the immune system is challenged by events like emotional stress, fatigue, or poor nutrition, the system may either go into a "hypo" or "hyper" state. In an underactive mode, invasion by harmful parasitic life becomes much more likely. When the system becomes hyperactive, like a "house-cleaning" service gone wild, the body attacks or overly "cleans" itself causing any one of a variety of what are called auto-immune disorders like rheumatoid arthritis and multiple sclerosis.

THE IMMUNE SYSTEM AND WINTER

To achieve a strong and balanced immune system and wellness throughout the stress symbolic "winter," we must first determine what it is about winter which allows the immune system to weaken and the beginning symptoms of the illness process to be set in motion. Once this concept is established, then the negative process can be reversed and health maintained or restored. Clearly, it does not take a scientific mind to conclude that somehow the colder temperatures must be involved. It is, however, narrow-minded to assume that a drop in the mercury is itself the sole cause of our weakened immune system. Common sense dictates that it takes something more all-encompassing than an occasional chill to isolate a strong physiology to a bedroom for recuperation. The root of the winter-illness relationship is the sustained low temperatures' negative affect on our positive lifestyle behaviors. When healthy lifestyle routines drop with the temperature, a process takes place which weakens our immune system.

Good examples of this phenomena can be cited in diet quality and exercise levels. Diet quality depreciates as the local growing season wanes. The vitamin, and enzyme value of the winter's supply of fruits and vegetables is usually far inferior to the value of those in the summer. Like this diminishing quality to dietary choices, our exercise routines also often slip when temperatures become uncomfortably low. With a decrease in essential exercise activity, muscle tone deteriorates, circulation slows, and nutrient absorption decreases. Without sufficient plant nutrients like Zinc and Vitamins A and C in the diet and adequate nutrient absorption from exercise and sunshine, the organs of the immune system weaken, their immune responses falter and the body becomes a likely candidate for infection. What should also be considered in this analysis is the winter's effect on our emotional state. When we are cooped up and inactive on a cold and dreary winter day, the unfavorable emotional state will inevitably adversely affect body chemistry and nutrient levels. Remember that the thymus, spleen, bone marrow, etc. need nutrients like all other body organs and when this supply becomes increasingly deficient or obstructed, their combined immune supporting functions invariably suffer and disease becomes imminent.

How and when do lifestyle changes, like those described during winter, result in infection or disease? The answer is determined by the following simplistic formula.

The Strength of the Genetic and Acquired Immune Response Minus the Nature and Sum of Lifestyle Violations = The Manifestation of Disease

When different lifestyle indiscretions combine, the ill effects of each on the immune system will be intensified. The sum equals more than the addition of the parts. The negative effect of an imbalanced diet and its low nutrient delivery to the immune system will be exacerbated when another lifestyle error like insufficient exercise or added emotional stress occurs. Whether the entire immune system matrix manifests this added strain as disease will be determined by the strength of both the genetically active and acquired immune systems. Even with many lifestyle indiscretions like smoking, drinking, etc., if by fate the genes are favorable and exposures minimal or innocuous, apparent symptoms of disease may be postponed or even never **noticed**. "Noticed" is emphasized here because, regardless of one's awareness of symptoms, added wear and tear from lifestyle faults will always progress to undermine health. When people follow abusive life patterns and pride themselves in never missing a day of work from sickness, it is usually not a contretemps when they "suddenly" discover they have a terminal cancer. Eventually, even with the best inherited make-up, the deferred penalty for lifestyle errors will be paid for by the genetically weakest body organ systems.

We can learn from the example of winter stress how important it is to maintain healthy lifestyle routines. Naturally we should always exclude or at least avoid unhealthy routines such as smoking, drinking, overeating, refined sugar consumption, etc. Granted this may require some education, ingenuity or extra enthusiasm, especially during the winter or a period of colder weather patterns, but like any other habit once established, it becomes increasingly simple to repeat. The following section will offer an overview of important lifestyle and adjunctive routines plus the fundamental educational groundwork necessary to understand and apply them. The major issue then left for us to overcome is psychological. As Somerset Maugham said, "The unfortunate thing about this world is that good habits are so much easier to give up than bad ones."

NATURE'S TOOLS

Philosophy

To learn to accept and use the following health routines, the best support we have is knowledge. No matter how valuable a system or tool is, if it is poorly understood, it is likely to go unappreciated and become discarded. To assist us in understanding nature's tools, we can thankfully rely upon the time-tested knowledge of naturopathy, the science of natural therapeutics. For purposes of this guidebook, trying my best to avoid misrepresentation, I have condensed this profound science into three of its most illuminating foundational principles. By acknowledging these, we can then begin to outline some natural therapeutics applicable to the immune system and appreciate why they work.

1. **The human body is a marvelous creation of nature. When the body's immune system becomes imbalanced and there is disease (usually resulting from our lifestyle errors), nature can be relied upon to provide the appropriate tools to restore and regenerate the health balance. These tools may be within the body's own homeostatic mechanisms or they may be found outside the body in the form of water, sunshine, herbs, fresh air, massage, etc.**

2. **The level of organ or system health is dependent upon both optimal absorption of**

nutrients and maximum elimination of metabolic toxins.

3. All body organs are unified and interconnected. To treat one system, all body organs and systems must be considered.

The Diet

To create a healthy immune system, nature's best tool is a consistent "balanced" and wholesome diet. Food really is the best medicine for not only the immune system but for every body system. A well designed diet insures that the second rule of naturopathy is achieved; that maximum nutrients are being consumed and absorbed and wastes are properly eliminated.

To reach the therapeutic function of diet, most of us need to make a change in our proportions of dietary constituents. Currently we eat too much animal proteins, fats, and refined carbohydrates. Foods richest in animal proteins and fats are meats and dairy products; refined carbohydrates are flour products like breads, pastries, and pastas. Unrefined carbohydrate and vegetable protein foods are fruits, vegetables, whole grains, beans, nuts and seeds. When the ratios tip in the favor of animal proteins, etc., the immune system is adversely affected. Why this particular dietary balance is weakening to the immune system will be summarized later in this guidebook, however, at this point what is important to recognize is that these animal protein, fat-rich refined carbohydrate foods demand the most from the digestive apparatus, create excess toxic build-up, and supply the least nutrient return to the immune system. Toxic build-up means the production and accumulation of harmful compounds like ammonia and bile salt degradation products which result from the digestive system's breaking down of respectively protein and fatty foods. These harmful compounds are then part of the food supply which instead of nourishing the immune system's organs, inevitably weaken or poison them. By eating more unrefined carbohydrate foods and decreasing concentrated animal foods, nutrient levels to the immune system will be optimized and potentially harmful digestive wastes will be accelerated in their transit.

The easiest and best way to counter the harmful protein-fat dietary habit is to increase rich dietary fiber foods, especially "whole" grains like cooked brown rice, millet, oats, etc. Contrary to popular opinion, a grain's fiber and nutrient effect cannot be optimally achieved by eating highly milled processed whole wheat or other "whole grain" breads. In these forms the fiber particle size is milled too fine, decreasing important water absorbability and leaving precious grain oils unnecessarily exposed to rancidity. There is one whole grain type bread which is an exception to the rule called Essene or Bible bread because of its ancient recipe. This naturally sweet high nutrient-fiber bread is produced from low-heated grain sprouts instead of rancid-prone flour. These breads can be found in your local health food store.

Besides eating more whole grains, keep in mind that the unrefined carbohydrate dietary balance is particularly tested in winter and that the problem of missing nutrients always needs to be addressed. In the summer, even if the central dietary item is animal protein, at least it is usually accompanied by balancing portions of fresh vegetables and corn. It is not coincidental that when there is a greater absence of fresh and appetizing produce that there is also an increase in sickness rates. To solve this potential nutrient depletion, become familiar with the fresh and dehydrated vegetables and fruits that are available in your area year-round like carrots, sprouts, apricots, seaweeds, etc., and learn how to tastefully prepare them. To assist you in the educational aspect of this process, there are a cornucopia of natural food cookbooks. Four of these that I highly recommend are the *McDougall Health Supporting Cookbook* by John and Mary McDougall, *Ten Talents* by Frank and Rosalie Hurd, *Moosewood Cookbook* by Mollie Katzen, and *Laurel's Kitchen* by Robertson, Flinders & Godfrey. By beginning to use the diet guidelines suggested in these cookbooks and in this guidebook, the quality of nourishment will improve and the immune system will strengthen.

Toxin Elimination

For optimal immunity, naturopathy also places great emphasis upon the elimination of systemic toxins which are generated from the combination of food breakdown, environmental exposure and general metabolism. Naturopathy teaches that if these systemic wastes are properly eliminated through the appropriate channels (the skin, lungs, urinary tract and large intestines), there is a minimized block to immune system response. On the other hand, if the body wastes are backed up in these channels and "recycled" instead of eliminated, the organs and response of the immune system will weaken from toxicity. A good nutrient and fiber-rich diet like the one described previously should help prevent this recycling process. Unfortunately though using a balanced meal plan of typical dietary foods alone is probably not enough. For too many years and through too many periods of emotional stress, seasonal change and concomitant lifestyle indiscretions, the eliminative channels have been improperly cared for or abused. The result is that the waste channels become stubbornly congested or obstructed and need added therapeutic attention.

How then should we attend to the different eliminative systems? To answer this question, we need to reflect upon the third principle of naturopathy that we outlined. This is simply that all the body's organs and systems are interdependent; the health and function of one system is reliant upon that of the others. In terms of the eliminative systems, if one system is unduly strained removing an excess of wastes, the others will inevitably take part of the load and reflect it. Common bad breath or "halitosis" exemplifies this. The putrid odor detected in the breath is really just excess toxic gases accumulated from other eliminative systems like the large intestines. The principle of eliminative system interconnectedness reminds us that if we want to restore optimal immune system response by relieving systemic wastes, we must use a "holistic" effort, which considers both individually and united all the body's waste channels.

The Skin and Kidneys

The skin is the body's largest eliminative organ. In the space of a postage stamp there are approximately 100 sweat glands, 15 sebaceous glands, 39 inches of blood vessels, and three million nerve cells. The skin requires even more attention during cold weather because the hundreds of thousands of pores are encumbered with more clothes and are therefore exposed to less nourishing air and light than in warmer seasons. Toxins are blocked from release and eventually block or interfere with skin nutrient absorption. A similar reaction occurs during a period of emotional stress. The end-result is a more sallow, dirty looking skin and a more toxic immune system. The following are four sample routines which will indirectly benefit the immune system because they help keep the skin waste channel nourished, open, and unencumbered.

1. **Dry Brush Massage**—At your local health food store there are special aloe fiber skin brushes which can invigorate the outer epidermal area and stimulate release of deeper "winter-stored" systemic toxins. Spend three to five minutes daily gently massaging the entire skin, being sure to rub in a circular motion from the extremities towards the heart.

2. **Ginger-Oatmeal Bath**—Like the aloe skin brush, ginger works to externally stimulate a sluggish skin system. Oatmeal is added for its soothing and nourishing properties to insure that the skin is not irritated and maintains its healthy lustre. With a filled tub, add at least one tablespoon of ground ginger with one-half cup of rolled oats. Try to take at least two Ginger-Oatmeal baths weekly.

3. **Improving Liquid Intake**—The skin is often called the "third kidney." By bettering the quality and in some cases quantity of

liquid intake, both the kidneys and skin are nourished and primed for better waste elimination. The macrobiotic instruction to drink when thirsty is the best common sense guide to determining the quantities of liquid consumed. Keep in mind, though, that this philosophy initially requires diligence and careful attention to our desires. Presently, many of us drink too little liquid because we have grown distant from our reflexes and instinctual cravings. Whatever the quantity, the type of liquid is important. A glass of spring water or a fresh glass of "Produce Juice" is obviously preferable to a cup of irritating coffee or cola. Produce juice is made with any one of a number of commercially available juice extractors like Champion and Acme which extract the vital juice of vegetables and fruits like carrot, celery, zucchini, beets, apples, peaches, etc. In consultations, I usually recommend 8 ounces daily of one's own favorite blend; carrot is usually used as the base. Different types of herbal teas can also serve as pleasurable alternatives to increase liquid intake. Good choices for a daily cup of tasteful tea are Peppermint, Chamomile, and Spearmint. These teas can also serve as a pleasant base for smaller amounts of more medicinal herbs like Pau Darco, Yarrow, Uva Ursi and Gravel Root. A sample therapeutic daily tea for the kidney-bladder could be one teaspoon of a blend of the first three with a one-half teaspoon blend of the latter four infused with eight ounces of spring water and a touch of honey. To a naturopath, these therapeutic herbs are considered "concentrated nutrient-rich foods." Different from drugs, which are often herb-extracted synthesized chemicals, whole herbs are a complex blend of nourishing and healing compounds. By learning how to use them, the direction of many body infirmities can be reversed. Herbalism, which is the age-old science of vegetative therapeutics and an integral part of naturopathy, is a source for many of the tools in this guidebook.

Following an "extended" liquid diet or what some may call fasting can also be an excellent lifestyle tool for skin and immune system health. Numerous scientific studies have demonstrated that fasting improves the immune system response and provides the digestive apparatus with a necessary therapeutic rest. When and how to fast is controversial and requires more of a detailed explanation than is possible in this guidebook. For general purposes though, when the appetite is naturally low and there is an excess of mucus or discharge, take at least 2-3 days to consume only fresh produce juice or low salt vegetable broths. Rest during this time, be moderate in the amounts of liquid consumed, and be sure to ease back slowly into the daily diet.

4. **Daily Exercise**—One famous naturopath wrote that the most important health routine to follow was to sweat daily through vigorous exercise. To some this means a walk around the block and to others it's a marathon run. In either case, the stimulation of exercise is important because it opens pores allowing toxins to leave and regenerating oxygen to enter.

5. **Adequate Rest**—Both exercise and rest are really health routines which could be equally applicable to the well-being of all waste channels. They are mentioned here in the context of skin health because this is where the benefit will be most noticeable. From adequate rest we gain nerve energy and vital force which give lustre to the skin and strength to all the organs of the immune system. Under the category of rest can be placed prayer, meditation and yoga. These activities refine and quiet mental activity beyond the benefits of sleep. As individual as our exercise routines are, the manner in which we rest is personal. Become aware of your own body's need for rest and the different routines which offer mental and physical quietness and then use discipline to apply them.

The Large Intestines

Of all the waste channels, the intestinal system is the least appreciated and most abused. The roots of this abuse run as deep as societal values. The large intestines and their elimination product are often the target for many culturally prevalent derogatory terms and personal attacks. Since eating and solid waste elimination is such a conspicuously important part of our daily lives and immune system health, and since there is this already pre-existing additional strain of disregard, this subject will be one of the focal points in this guidebook. If we were as willing to nurture and beautify our intestinal tract as we are our skin, this added attention would be unnecessary.

The intestinal waste channel can help create the nadir point of immune system health through a process popularly called "auto-intoxication" which means self-poisoning. Even though most lay writings equate this term with intestinal malfunction, it should be remembered that all the waste channels possess the same adverse potential. By appreciating at least the basics of this process as it occurs in the large intestine, concern will hopefully mount to improve the diet and begin a regenerative routine. The following is a description of the chain of events that connect a distressed intestines to a poisoned immune system. The reader should be aware that much more attention could be given to this topic to do it justice and that the discussion herein is intended as a summary or introduction.

The scenario most likely to create auto-intoxication is the consumption of a low nutrient, deficient fiber, high animal protein, fatty food diet under added environmental or internal stress. To manifest this potential condition, imagine a fast-food, fat-dripping hamburger with deep fried french fries and a shake as a regular dietary item. The added environmental or internal stresses could be the restaurant itself, a seasonal change, low vitality from inadequate exercise or a detrimental emotional experience. All of these stress factors magnify the dangerous effects of dietary abuse by weakening the essential matrix of digestive functioning. The following charts the path of this typical gastronomic event.

The meal is poorly masticated because it is deficient in fiber. Salivary moisture and starch digesting enzymes are deficient. Excess starch reaches the stomach, absorbing protein-digesting stomach acids. The meat proteins are therefore left improperly digested. When the meal reaches the small intestines, there is inadequate acid or too high a pH to sufficiently stimulate appropriate amounts of acid-buffering and digestant pancreatic enzymes. The result is hyperacidic exposure leading to an ulcer-prone small intestine and poorly digested starches and proteins. The meat and shake's high fat content intensifies the meal's harm by slowing stomach digestion and causing a rush of excess irritating bile acids for prolonged tissue exposure. Once the food reaches the last portion of the small intestines, the real witches cauldron effect takes place. While whatever available nutrients are being extracted and absorbed, the irritating undigested food mass is being prepared for its ill-fated meeting with the "intestinal flora." The intestinal flora is a mass of approximately thirty-five trillion microbes, which when exposed to undigested material, does its own "digesting." If this pattern of bacteria is harmful and the diet is rich in animal proteins, fats, and refined carbohydrates, which is the common case in our culture, the food breakdown by bacteria results in "putrefaction" or food rotting. Putrefaction is similar to the phenomenon that takes place in a container of milk or meat if it has been left in a warm spot or kept too long. There is a major difference though between this and what occurs in the human physiology. When a milk container is rotten, it is discarded; when the putrefied food is in the human large intestines, it is often either ignored or considered humorous. Regardless of our reaction to this problem, the adverse nature to this internal process is well documented in medical literature. Besides the ammonia and carcinogenic bile salt degradation products which are shown to be produced from protein-fat metabolism, additional poisonous incomplete protein breakdown products (IPBs) like cadaverine and putrescine are generated from putrefaction. The blend of these products then join and react as an added unremitting irritation to our delicate absorptive intestinal lining. When these (IPBs) inevitably enter the blood stream, they are treated as "foreign bodies" and thusly place a constant demand upon and weaken the immune system. Over an extended period of time, this type of diet inevitably causes inflammation and mucus discharge to become a constant state as the body's immune system uses all its resources to protect itself from life-threatening injury. As the immune system weakens, everything from a worsening allergy to a silent unrestricted cancer growth becomes a greater possibility.

In summation, there are two basic points to be extracted from this short analysis. The first is that there is a relationship between one's immune state and the condition of the intestinal tract. The second is that dietary abuse and its detrimental digestive consequences systemically affect every body system. Even if blatant illnesses like ulcers and cancer do not result from the strained tissues and intestinal toxins, the added stress on the digestive waste channel, from diet indiscretions like the one described, can be blamed for much of the malaise from which untold numbers of us suffer.

To reverse the life-damaging process of intestinal auto-intoxication, besides applying the healthy diet and lifestyle regimes, a more specific intestinal "tune-up" program can be followed which specifically deals with the problem of accumulated intestinal toxins and weakened degenerated tissues. An intestinal "tune-up" can be healthfully initiated for one month at the beginning of each season. The following is a description of one such effective and well-researched program using herbs and other nourishing food supplements. If these blends cannot be found, contact your trained herbalist, nutrition counselor, or doctor for good substitute blends. To simplify this search, be sure to use a combination of nourishing fiber from the mucilage an gum groups with a high potency, implantable beneficial microbial strain. The vegetable Okra is of particular value as a source for nourishing and soothing fiber. To replace the combinations described as 2-4 respectively, use a blend of herbs titled carminatives, cholagogues, and laxatives. The value of the blends suggested here is that they are gentle and properly balanced. The (A) after each herb symbolizes the active or principal agent, the (B) represents a balancer or synergistic herb. The number equals the suggested proportions. With your counselor's and manufacturer's guidelines, follow as similar a routine as possible to the one outlined. Fortunately, there are a number of high quality brands available which accomplish these basic requirements.

Whatever the program brand though, be aware that the path to good health can sometimes be rocky and may require extra care. This is especially true in the first few weeks. When there are years of neglect, sometimes the initial process of restoration can cause an intensification of the uncomfortable symptoms trying to be corrected. One way to better understand this unpleasant side to restoration is to use an analogy of seeing a dentist. Filling cavities and cleaning the teeth is sometimes uncomfortable but clearly it is vital to dental health. So too, cleansing and building the solid eliminative system requires some trying times. During this period there may be some cramping, excess gas expulsion and embarrassment, however considering the long term benefits, these are minimal concerns. Be aware that optimal health is a state which requires dedication and sometimes hard work; the patent tonics that promise overnight vitality and instant health are misleading and potentially harmful. This heeding should also be kept in mind when we face a "cold" or fever and the temptation for "12 hour relief." Naturopathy teaches that higher body temperatures and excess mucus should not be suppressed because they are natural mechanisms for toxin removal. When these symptoms of normal immune system functioning are repressed instead of assisted, toxins move deeper and cause more serious future problems. If you are ill, be sure to consult and carefully plan with your physician before beginning any new routines. This is especially true if you are using prescription drugs. Some herbs and drugs do not mix well and can cause potentially adverse reactions.

Item 1

A Bio-Culture of three strains of bacteria, Lactobacillus acidophilus, Streptococcus faecium and Bifidus.

The supplementation with this product(s) replaces and inhibits the activity of harmful microbial strains at the point where food and bacteria meet. By doing this, food residues will be less likely to rot and proper digestive mechanics can be restored. This product can be thought of as a concentrate of the good properties of yogurt. The benefits of using this supplement in addition to or instead of yogurt are that these "good" bacteria can flourish in the intestinal tract and that their numbers are therapeutically high. The Streptococcus faecium strain, despite its awful sounding name, is particularly valuable. Its acid and heat resistant properties allow it to better implant in the large intestine and compete with the more virulent microbial populations. The following summarizes the Bio-Culture's documented effects:

1. Attracts moisture to the intestines, softening stools and diluting toxins.
2. Neutralizes intestinal carcinogenic enzyme activity.
3. Produces necessary B vitamins and digestive enzymes.
4. Performs natural antibiotic functions.

Suggested Use: Take 4-500 mg. capsules or one-half teaspoon three times daily for the first two weeks on an empty stomach with 4-8 ozs. of juice or spring water. Daily dosage during this period should be at least fifteen billion cells. After the initial two week period, take once daily on an empty stomach. This routine can be followed year-round. If the immune system is under particular stress, or if dairy products are included in the diet, increase to the initial dosage.

Combination 1:

Texan Biodynamic Okra (A) 3   Slippery Elm Bark (A) 3
Marshmallow Root(A) 2   Licorice (B) 1
Chlorella (B) 1   Wheat grass (B) 1
Jamaican Ginger (B) 1

The herbs in this blend provide valuable cleansing and nourishing fiber groups for general digestive health and better nutrient absorption. Unlike many bulk-forming preparations, this combination is rich in nutrients and can help rebuild weakened and irritated tissues.

Suggested Use: Take 3 capsules or 1/2 tsp. powder daily with juice or water on an empty stomach. It is best to take this daily dosage one of the times the "bioculture" is used. The "bioculture" converts the fiber in this blend into beneficial therapeutic products for gastro-intestinal health. This routine can be followed year-round.

Combination 2:

Peppermint 3	Papaya Leaf 2
Cloves 2	Jamaican Ginger 1
Gentian 2	Cayenne 1/2
Fennel 1	

All the herbs in this blend are both active principals (A) and balancers(B).

Historically these herbs are renowned for stimulating normal gastric protein digestion and dispelling toxic gases. This blend offers an alternative to supplementing the diet with concentrated digestive enzymes which some authorities suspect may create dependency.

Suggested Use: Take 2 capsules or 20 extract drops with 4-8 ozs. of spring water five minutes prior to eating a high protein meal. After the one month program is completed, this blend can be valuable for use during periods of stress or irregular diet patterns.

Combination 3:

Goldenseal (A) 3	Gentian (B) 1
Barberry (A) 3	Wild Yam (A) 2
Prickly Ash (A) 1	Mullein (B) 1
Alfalfa (B) 1	

Combination 4:

Senna Pods (A) (Not leaf) 3	Cascara Sagrada (A) 3
Barberry (B) 2	Mullein (B) 1
Cloves (B) 2	Licorice(B) 1

Combinations 3 & 4 both stimulate digestive secretions and particularly the activity of the liver, gall bladder, pancreas and large intestine. The primary aim of Combination 3 is to promote activity in a sluggish and toxic liver, gall bladder, and pancreas. Combination 4 demonstrates its most pronounced activity on large intestinal functioning. It assists in the initial stage of removal of impactions or obstructive waste material.

Suggested Use: Combinations 3 & 4 should only be used for a two week period at the beginning of the eliminative health program. They may also be used briefly during times of tension or stress if bowel function seems to become congested. Combination 4 will be more stimulating in a powder or capsule form than in a liquid tincture. Neither combination should be used during pregnancy or without the advice of a physician if there has been a history of bowel disturbances. Experiences with these blends will vary with the individual, so begin with a minimum amount, like one capsule or ten drops of each with 4-8 ozs. of spring water, and increase slowly until some stimulation of eliminative behavior is observed.

Lungs

It is appropriate to touch upon the lung system at this time. Wastes obstructed here will also return to the blood stream and weaken immunity. To restore and heal this waste channel, naturopathy places great emphasis upon the importance of fresh air and deep breathing. In modern city life, this means trying to take the time daily for a brisk walk or jog through a park trail or down a quiet street. One advantage of winter time is that a walk's briskness comes naturally. The following are two sample naturopathic routines helpful for lung health.

1. Moist Chest Packs and Steam Inhalations
    Appropriate herbs for this are Jamaican Ginger, Eucalyptus and Peppermint. While bathing, use a cotton cloth or small towel soaked in a combination of these teas. Wrap it around the chest while occasionally applying hot water in order to maintain the warm temperature and steam for 15-20 minutes. At the end of the moist chest pack and before leaving the

bath, cover the forehead and chest with a cool cloth for 30 seconds to one minute.

2. Herbal Teas

Equal parts of Osha, Fenugreek, Echinacea, Mullein, Wild Cherry, Licorice and Chickweed combined makes a healthful lung tea which assists in toxin removal. When mucus seems to be accumulating, make 3 cups of this tea and sip it throughout the day. For convenience and better nutrient absorption, many of these herbs are available in extract form. As a general recommendation, use 30 drops of extract for each cup of tea.

Herbal Support

Once the "channels of elimination" are attended to and cleaned, specific food supplements can be recommended to support the immune system. These agents provide "concentrated" nourishment to strengthen the immune system and assist in stimulating normal eliminative functioning. The following six are good examples of the best known throughout naturopathic literature. Since all six of these are nutrient-rich non-irritating products, their use can be recommended year-round. In the enthusiasm for re-discovering health, you do not need to feel obliged to use all these products, simply begin to experiment with the ones that appeal to you most.

1. **Garlic**—Probably more than any other single food, this herb can help form a barrier between you and disease. Reputed for its antibiotic and stimulating features since time immemorial, garlic's sulfur-rich properties make it one of nature's best immune system therapeutics.

Suggested Use: It is preferable to eat at least one clove fresh daily. A good way to add garlic to the diet is to squeeze it over a fresh salad with lemon and apple cider vinegar. If odor is a concern, chew on the spice herb called cloves or fresh parsley afterwards. If this is still not satisfactory, take one of the commercial deodorized non-oil encapsulated brands.

2. **Royal Jelly**—Royal Jelly is a bee secretion produced by worker bees to solely nourish and "create" a queen bee. From this phenomenal substance, an average female worker is transformed into a queen and outlives her workers by twenty-fold. An analysis of Royal Jelly's nutrients reveals a wide range of nutrients. It is particularly rich in the B vitamin pantothenic acid which can help restore and support a weakened stress response system. In China, Royal Jelly is renowned for its strengthening properties and is particularly suggested for its support to the reproductive system.

Suggested Use: Take one 200 mg. Fresh Royal Jelly capsule daily.

3. **Bee Pollen**—Research conducted by biologists and botanists like Dr. Nicolai Tsitsin and Dr. Emil Chauvin has demonstrated that Bee Pollen can be a vital health tool for well-being throughout periods of stress. The principle reason for this supportive influence is its high nutrient and enzyme value, which according to Dr. Naum Joirisch of the Academy of Science, allows it to regenerate the system and slow the aging process. A key element in choosing a quality bee pollen is the environment from which the pollen is collected. Few people realize that pollen, even though a "super-food," is also an accurate "environmental-pollutant" indicator. To avoid this potential problem, one national region, with Montana as the key state, called the "Big Sky," offers the healthiest, purest, uncontaminated pollen.

Suggested Use: Take one teaspoon or six 500 mg. capsules daily. Before reaching this daily recommended dosage, increment very slowly to avoid potential allergic reactions. This means to take 1 granule on first day, 2 the next day, etc. until the desired dosage is attained. The same procedure should be followed with the capsules. Empty the capsule and fill with only a few granules, exercising care to increase a little each day. If there is a sensitivity, it usually manifests as a throat scratchiness or skin-itching.

4. **Panax Ginsengs**—Probably more than any other single food supplement, Ginseng (Panax species) has earned a reputation as an adaptogen. This means that through its constitutents of nutrients and plant compounds called ginsenosides, it increases the body's flexibility to adapt to internal stress and changing environmental conditions that affect our immunity.

Suggested Use: There are almost as many different opinions about how and when to use ginseng as there are herbalists. The truth to ginseng usage lies within each individual. To discover your own best utilization of this herb, experiment in small amounts with different varieties like the Chinese "Red and White" or Wild American Panax forms. Each will have its own qualities and potencies. As a general recommendation, take a manufacturer's suggested dose twice weekly and try to combine it with a tea of ground ginger and licorice. These two herbs help balance any potential excess stimulation of the bodily energy system, called Chi in the Orient, by the Panax species.

5. **Wheat Grass Juice (Powdered)**—The dried extracted juice of the green wheat grass is a rich source of readily assimilable Beta-Carotene, Vitamins K and C, calcium, and blood cleansing chlorophyll. University research has shown that the domestic organically grown wheat grass juice source, which allows for the manifestation of the full jointing wheat growth phase, is at least four times as high in important nutrients like chlorophyll and calcium as are the rapid growth home cultivated produced juices.

Suggested Use: Take three 500 mg. capsules daily on an empty stomach with spring water. This will be equivalent to slightly more than 1 oz. of fresh juice.

6. **Evening Primrose Oil**—It is well accepted amongst the scientific community that breast-fed infants demonstrate superior immune responses. One theory often offered to help explain this positive difference is that breast milk stimulates the production of certain beneficial forms of microbial life like the bifidus strain we previously discussed. These then successfully compete with harmful or parasitic strains. Another even more intriguing theory, which is probably not exclusive of the first, is that human breast milk is one of nature's rare sources of a compound called dihomo-gammalinolenic acid (DGLA) which the infant's body can convert into a specific prostaglandin (PG) called PGE 1. Medical research suggests that PGE 1 can help play a preventive or curative role in a host of potential immune system disorders ranging from multiple sclerosis and cancer to hyperactivity and premenstrual stress syndrome (PMS). The relationship between the therapeutic effect of mother's milk and Evening Primrose Oil is that Evening Primrose Oil is a rare natural source of gamma-linolenic acid (GLA), a precursor of (DGLA) from which the body can manufacture PGE 1. Evening Primrose Oil can therefore provide many of the immune supportive benefits associated with mother's milk. It should be mentioned that among the known blockers to the body's ultimate formation of PGE 1 are processed vegetable oils, saturated fats, and a lack of vitamins B6 and minerals zinc and magnesium.

Suggested Use: Take two 500 mg. capsules daily.

There are five other items or blends (lettered A, B, C, D, E) which are specifically useful during period of intense immune system stress.

Combination A:

Wild American Ginseng (20 yr. root) (A2)
Saw Palmetto (A2)
Parsley Root (A1)
Cascara Sagrada (A1)

Gentian (B1)
Dandelion Root(A2)
Uva Ursi (A2)
Cayenne (B1/2)

Combination B:

Wild American Ginseng (20 yr. root) (A3)
Gentian (B2)
Peppermint (B3)

Wild Yam (A2)
Saw Palmetto (A2)

When the body is confronted with the classic stress "fight or flight" response, the blood sugar levels must rise to the demand. When the blood sugar levels fail to properly respond or sustain long term abuse, the immune system's integrity becomes challenged. Blend A is a combination of herbs historically used to help support strained pancreatic blood sugar metabolism. Blend B, according to its historical usage, helps support the stress-responding adrenal glands. The principal agent responsible for the stress support effect in both these combinations is a 20 yr. Wild American Ginseng root (Panax quinquefolium). Wild American Ginseng is particularly high in ginsenosides which assist the body's response to stress. A 20 year wild root is recommended because the long maturation time allows the herb to draw the highest nutrient and therapeutic value possible from the soil. Some Oriental herbalists do not recommend using Panax Ginseng when there is a flu-type illness because of its stimulating properties, therefore use discretion during this time.

Suggested Use: The same suggestions apply to both blends. Take two 500 mg capsules or 20 drops of the extract with 4-8 ozs. of spring water one hour after eating a meal. These combinations should be used whenever the body seems to be experiencing inordinate stress. There are some stimulating herbs in these blends so it is best to only use for a limited period of time (2-3 months).

Item C:
Pure Bee Propolis
Bee Propolis is a resinous substance which bees collect and form to help protect the hive from infection. Not surprisingly, a similar antibiotic phenomena is noticed when this product is supplemented in the human diet.

Suggested Use: Take two 500 mg capsules four times daily with 4-8 ozs. of spring water. on an empty stomach at the first signs of infection, along with the recommended dietary addition of Combination D. Use care with this and items D and E to not use during infection as a replacement for a doctor's care.

Item D:
Echinacea angustifolia
Echinacea represents one of nature's best herbs to help the immune system fight infection. Currently medical science is aware of at least three important constituents to this herb; These are echinacin B, (Z)-1, 8-pentadecadiene, and echinacoside. Respectively these principles have been shown to possess the following properties; Wound-healing, anti-tumor and bacteriostatic.

Suggested Use: Take two 500 mg. capsules or 20 extract drops three times daily at the first signs of infection.

Combination E:

Echinacea angustifolia (A2)	Pau Darco (A2)
Siberian Ginseng (B1)	Myrrh (A1)
Cayenne (B1/2)	Black Walnut (A1)
Goldenseal (A2)	Propolis (A1)
Chlorella (B1)	L. Acidophilus (A200 million)
Streptococcus faecium (SF) (A200 million)	
Ligustrum (A2)	Astragalus (A2)

Combination E is a synergistic sampling of nature's tools to help the immune system fight an actual illness. Besides containing

Propolis and Echinacea, there are 11 other compounds which accentuate and expand the combination's therapeutic range. There are two herbs that are renowned in Chinese Herbalism. These herbs are Astragalus membranaceus and Ligustrum lucidum and are detailed in the excellent book by Ron Teeguarden, *Chinese Tonic Herbs*. An overview of preliminary laboratory findings on Astragulus and Ligustrum hints at the great therapeutic potential that lies in many of our common herbs. Research performed by the National Cancer Institute and five other cancer research institutes have concluded that supplementation with the Astragalus and Ligustrum herbs was responsible for the restoration in immune functions in 90% of the cancer patients studied. In other research Astragalus was found to increase natural interferon production and reduce the so-called T-suppressor cells which inhibit one's immune response. Because of findings like these, the researchers are proposing applications for Astragalus and Ligustrum in other immune disorders like AIDS. With cases like these being reported for hundreds of different common herbs, it is easy to appreciate the truth behind Ralph Waldo Emerson's definition of a weed. "Weed—a plant whose virtues have not yet been discovered."

Suggested Use: Take two 500 mg. capsules twice daily with 4-8 ozs. of spring water on an empty stomach during a period of environmental or internal stress. At the first signs of infection follow the same routine as above except dose three times daily.

EPILOGUE

In closing, it would be remiss to not remind the reader of an underlying naturopathic principle that, independent of season, most profoundly affects our immunity; this is the connection of our mental-emotional-spiritual state to our physical well-being. Even though herbs and water applications, etc. can be soothing and even regenerating to our immune system and physical body, there is no naturopathic treatment I am aware of, other than the warmth of love, which can truly mend the repercussions of a "broken heart." We should not forget that if negative emotions like hurt or anger are allowed to be sublimated and fester, there will be a gradual, daily degeneration of the genetically weakest "disease-prone" physical body organs. The following traditional story of two monks accentuates the importance of the mind-body relationship.

Two monks with vows of celibacy were approached by a woman for assistance to cross the river. The first monk refused to aid the woman because of his holy vows. The second monk obliged, and carried the well-dressed woman across the stream. After a week had passed, the first monk angrily challenged the second on his seeming transgression. The second monk wisely retorted, "I carried the woman for five minutes, you have carried her for seven days." No matter how valuable our routine, diet or philosophy, in our quest for health, we should try not to forget that happiness is the highest objective.

Good Health To All

SUGGESTED READING AND REFERENCES

Arehart-Treichel, Joan. *Immunity—How Our Bodies Resist Disease.* New York: Holiday House, 1976

Ballentine, M.D., Rudolph. *Diet & Nutrition—A Holistic Approach.* Honesdale, PA: Himalayan International Institutie, 1982

Burkitt, Denis P. *Colonic-Rectal Cancer: Fiber and Other Dietary Factors.* Am J Clin Nutr 31: S 58- S 64, 1978

Goldin, B.R., and S. L. Gorbach. *The Relationship Between Diet and Rat Fecal Bacterial Enzymes Implicated in Colon Cancer.* J Natl Cancer Inst. 57:371, 1976, and *The Effect of Milk and Lactobacillus Feeding on Human Intestinal Bacterial Enzyme Activity.* Am J Clin. Nutr 39: May 1984, pp 756-61

Grieve, M. *A Modern Herbal: Vols 1 & 2.* New York: Dover Publications, 1971

Griggs, Barbara. *Green Pharmacy—A History of Herbal Medicine.* New York:Methuen, 1981

Hare, Caspari, Rusby. *The National Standard Dispensatory,* 1905

Harriman, Sarah. *The Book of Ginseng.* New York: Pyramid Books, 1975

Heinerman, John. *The Science of Herbal Medicine.* Orem, Utah: Bi-World, 1979

Hoffman, David. *The Holistic Herbal*. Findhorn:Findhorn Press, 1983

Jensen D.C., Bernard. *Nature Has A Remedy*. Self Published:Escondido, CA, 1981

McDougall, M.D., John A., *The McDougall Plan*. Piscataway, N.Y.: New Century Publishers, 1983

Mendelsohn, M.D., Robert. *Confessions of a Medical Heretic*. New York: Warner Books, 1980

W.E.C. Moore, Ph.D., E.P. Cato, M.S., and L.V. Holdeman, Ph.D., *Some Current Concepts in Intestinal Bacteriology*, Am J Clin Nutr 31:S33-S42.1978

Ohsawa, George. *Macrobiotics: An Invitation To Health And Happiness*. Oroville, CA:Ohsawa Macrobiotic Foundation, 1984

Santillo, Humbart. *Natural Healing with Herbs*. Prescott Valley, AZ:Hohm Press, 1984

Selye, Hans. *The Stress of Life* , New York:McGraw Hill, 1978

Shahani, K. Ayebo, A.D. *Role of Dietary Lactobacilli in Gastrointestinal Microecology*, Am J Clin Nutr, Nov. 1980 pp 2448-2457

Shelton, Herbert M. *Fasting Can Save Your Life*. Bridgeport, CT:Natural Hygiene, 1978

Teeguarden, Ron. *Chinese Tonic Herbs*. New York: Japan Publications. Jan 1985

Tucker, D and Colleagues, *Dietary Fiber and Personality Factors as Determinants of Stool Output.* Gastroenterology 1981; 81:879-83

U.S. Dept. of Health and Human Services—Public Health Service. *Immunology—Its Role in Health and Disease.* NIH Publication No. 80-940, 1980.

Visek, W.J. *Diet and Cell Growth Modulation by Ammonia.* Am J Clin Nutr. 31:S 216-S, 220, 1978

Vogel, A. *Swiss Nature Doctor.* Teufen AR, Switzerland, 1980

Wilen, Joan, Wilen, Lydia. *Chicken Soup & Other Folk Remedies.* New York:Ballantine Books, 1984